HERBAL REMEDIES AND NATURAL MEDICINE FOR BEGINNERS

By Smith J. Offor

Table of Contents

Introduction

Herbal Treatments for Novices

Even the supplement industry, which generates 31 billion dollars annually, is a trillion-dollar industry, as are the medical and pharmaceutical sectors. They're not making this much money by curing people's illnesses, so for what?

Drugs are not what herbals are

When using an herbal remedy, you must use caution. Nutritional supplements include herbal remedies. They aren't pharmaceuticals. The following are some things to be aware of regarding herbal remedies:

- Herbals are not subject to the same regulations as medications.

- Prior to sale, herbal products do not require strict testing.

- Herbal remedies might not function as promised.

- Any authority does not need to approve labels. The quantity of an ingredient might not be listed correctly

- There is a chance that some herbal remedies include additives or contaminants that are not disclosed on the label

Natural Does Not Equal Safe

A lot of people believe that using plants instead of medications is safer for treating illness. Plants have long been used in folk medicine by humans. Consequently, it is simple to understand the appeal. But "natural" does not equate to secure. Some herbal remedies can interact with other medications or be toxic in high doses if not taken as prescribed. Several could also have negative effects.

Here are a few instances:

Herb kava is used to treat menopause symptoms, anxiety, insomnia, and other conditions. Studies suggest that it might help with anxiety. However, kava can seriously harm the liver. There is a warning against using it from the FDA.

St. For mild to moderate depression, John's Wort might be effective. Antidepressants, birth control pills, and other medications may interact with it.

Additionally, it may result in adverse effects like anxiety and upset stomach.

To treat erectile dysfunction, yohimbe bark is used.

Other negative effects of the bark include anxiety, elevated blood pressure, and increased heart rate.

It may interact with specific antidepressant medications. It can be dangerous to take it frequently or in large doses.

The effectiveness of some herbal remedies for their intended uses has, of course, been tested. Many are also quite safe, but the term "natural" does not necessarily indicate which products are safe or unsafe.

How to Select and Utilize Herbal Treatments Safely

Some herbal remedies can improve your health and make you feel better. But you must practice wise consumer behavior. When selecting herbal remedies, remember these suggestions.

Examine the product's claims in great detail. Such claims are warning signs: Are they made about the product? Is it a "miracle" pill that "melts away" fat? Does it work faster than standard treatment? Is it a well-kept secret that your doctor and the drug companies don't want you to know? It's probably not true if something seems too good to be true.

Recall that "real-life stories" are not valid sources of evidence. Real-life examples are frequently used to promote products.

5

Even if the provider of the quote provided it, there is no guarantee that other customers will experience the same outcomes.

Consult your provider before utilizing a product.

Ask them what they think. The product's safety, likelihood of effectiveness, risks, potential for drug interactions, and ability to affect your treatment are all factors to consider.

Purchase only from businesses whose products are marked with certification, such as "USP Verified" or "ConsumerLab Approved Quality.". With these certifications, businesses pledge to test their products' quality and purity.

If you are over 65 years old, you should not use or give herbal supplements to children:

Consult your provider initially.

If you take any medications, avoid using herbal remedies without first consulting your doctor.

If you are expecting or nursing a baby, avoid using them.

When having surgery, avoid using them.

Always disclose to your healthcare provider what herbal remedies you take. They may have an impact on the medications you take as well as any medical treatments.

Further publications to consult

1. James Green's manual for herbal medicine makers

Comprehensive instructions for making herbal medicines, such as tinctures, ointments, salves, etc.

This foray into making medicine should be accompanied by a good deal of philosophical waxing.

2. RichoCech's Making Plant Medicine

Targeting those who grow their own herbs.

3. Written by Michael Moore, Herbal MateriaMedica

Contains a succinct description of the main medicinal plants, including preferred media, strengths, typical dosage ranges, potential side effects, and ecological status.

When determining the right ratios and dosages for your tinctures, you can refer to this resource with ease.

The Southwest School of Botanical Medicine website offers free access to this resource.

An extensive but very user-friendly manual for creating medications that includes the authors' favorite formulas. Contains suggested applications and dosages for a wide range of herbs.

9

Some Recommended literature on Herbal Remedies for Women, Children, And Infants.

1. Botanical Medicine for Women's Health, by Aviva Romm

An extensive source of traditional and modern knowledge about medical and herbal treatments for problems with women's health. This is the most sophisticated and comprehensive book on the topic, and it is written with the healthcare professional in mind.

2. By Rosemary Gladstar, "Herbal Healing for Women: Easy Home Remedies for All Ages."

engaging and comprehensive medical literature. On a three-month trip to Central America, Juliet only had this one book with her, and she never got bored reading it. Many formulas and recipes make information very available.

3. The Natural Pregnancy Book by Aviva Romm includes information on herbs, diet, and other holistic options.

Follows a woman's journey from conception to delivery and describes herbs that can support and maintain a healthy pregnancy as well as those you should avoid while you're pregnant.

4. Aviva Romm's third edition of The Natural Pregnancy Book: Your

Complete Guide to a Safe, Organic Pregnancy and Childbirth with Herbs, Nutrition, and Other Holistic Options. Focuses on the typical health problems that affect kids, from babies to pre-adolescents.

5. Mary Bove's Natural Healing Encyclopedia for Kids & Infants

A comprehensive, simple-to-follow manual for keeping kids healthy that covers diet, supplements, and herbal remedies. With a focus on the immune system, it offers advice and recipes for more than 50 common ailments.

Herbal medications

Drugs classified as herbal are those whose active components are derived from plant materials like leaves, roots, or flowers. However, just because something is "natural" doesn't necessarily mean it's safe for you to consume it.

Herbal medicines have an impact on the body in a similar way to conventional drugs, and if used improperly, they may even be harmful.

Therefore, they ought to be used with the same caution and deference as traditional medications.

Inform your doctor or pharmacist right away if you plan to have surgery, have a health consultation, or take any herbal medications.

Potential problems with herbal remedies.

Be aware of the following if you currently use or intend to use any herbal medications.

If you also take other medications, they could become problematic. They might reduce the effectiveness of the other medication or result in unanticipated side effects.

After taking an herbal medicine, you might have a negative reaction or experience side effects.

All herbal medications are not governed.

There is no requirement for a license to prepare medications specifically for a single person, and there may be no regulations governing medications made outside of the UK.

The evidence supporting the efficacy of herbal medicines is typically very scant. They may be useful to some people, but often their use is based more on custom than on scientific study.

The use of herbal medications should be avoided by a few specific demographic groups.

Who should stay away from herbal remedies
The following people shouldn't use an herbal remedy:

- Individuals who also take other medications, such as combined pills or hormonal contraceptives.

- People with severe medical conditions, like kidney or liver disease.

- Individuals who will undergo surgery.

- Women in pregnancy or who are nursing.

- Elderly people.

- Children – Just like with conventional medications, herbal medications should be stored out of the sight and reach of young children.

- If you belong to one of these categories, consult your physician or pharmacist for guidance before attempting an herbal remedy.

Surgery and herbal remedies

Before having surgery, it's crucial to let your doctor know if you take any herbal medications.

The reason for this is:

- Some herbal remedies may interact with anesthesia and other medications taken prior to, during, or after procedures.
- Some herbal remedies may affect blood pressure and blood clotting, which could increase the risk of bleeding during or following surgery.

- Therefore, in the weeks leading up to your operation, your doctor might advise you to stop taking any herbal supplements.

What to search for when purchasing a herbal remedy

If you want to try an herbal remedy, look for the traditional herbal registration (THR) marking on the product packaging.

This indicates that the medication meets high standards for manufacturing, safety, and the provision of usage instructions.

But bear in mind that:

THR products are intended to treat conditions like coughs, colds, and general aches and pains that can be treated without a doctor's assistance.

THR products may be dangerous if used for more severe conditions, especially if you delay seeking medical attention.

 In spite of claims to the contrary, the efficacy of THR products has not been established.

The presence of a THR label does not guarantee that a product can be used by anyone without any risks.

THR-registered products are available at the neighborhood pharmacy, grocery store, and health store.

Risks involved in ordering herbal medicine by mail or online.

• The likelihood of receiving fake, subpar, illegal, or contaminated medication increases when ordering prescription drugs online or by mail.

• Non-UK licensed herbal medications may not be subject to regulation.

• They could be counterfeit versions of licensed drugs produced in unlicensed facilities without quality control.

• Some websites may look legitimate even though they are fronted by people impersonating doctors or pharmacists.

• Additionally, herbal products purchased online may contain harmful and illegal ingredients.

There is a list of prohibited and restricted herbal ingredients on the GOV.

It's best to avoid products like herbal weight-loss supplements and those that claim to improve sexual performance.

This is because it has been found that they contain dangerous ingredients—like pharmaceutical ones that aren't listed on the label—that are dangerous.

Side effects information

You can report any adverse effect or side effect from a herbal medicine using the Yellow Card Scheme, which is run by the Medicines and Healthcare products Regulatory Agency (MHRA).

This can help the MHRA identify any new risks or side effects associated with medications, including herbal remedies.

If: You should report any negative effects or side effects.

You speculate that the prescription medication or herbal supplement you were taking may have contributed to the side effect or unfavorable reaction.

When you take multiple prescription medications or herbal remedies, the side effect occurs.

In particular, if the herbal remedy has a brand name or manufacturer, it's critical to provide as much information as you can.

In the past, Yellow Card reports have been used to draw attention to the dangers of using unlicensed Ayurvedic and traditional Chinese medicines that contain dangerous elements like mercury, lead, and arsenic as well as interactions between St. John's wort and various medicines.

The Foundations of Healing Herbs

Herbal remedies have been used for thousands of years in various traditional medical procedures all over the world. Many of these serve as inspiration for contemporary medications that use comparable active ingredients. But for those of us who prefer a more natural, holistic approach to our health, the real thing is usually the better option.

If you want to increase the variety of medicinal herbs you already have at home and are just getting started with herbal medicine, this beginner's guide is perfect for you.

The top ten herbs to keep on hand will be discussed, with an emphasis on those that have a variety of positive effects on your health and well-being.

1. The color green tea.

One of our top picks for promoting overall health is green tea. Due to its high antioxidant content, green tea is excellent for lowering blood pressure, reducing inflammation, enhancing brain function, bolstering our immune systems, and even helping with weight loss.

2. Ashwagandha.

Without ashwagandha, another medicinal herb, we couldn't survive. Ayurveda's most important herb, ashwagandha, helps the body and mind cope with stress and anxiety. Additionally, it enhances our capacity for concentration and focus, as well as our capacity for athletic performance and sleep quality.

3. Liquorice.

Lovely liquorice, a great herb to have on hand for liver protection, digestion calming, and immune system support. The sweetness of this calming herb reduces menopausal hot flashes and soothes sore throats and coughs.

4. Chamomile.

Our go-to herb of choice for calming the nervous system and helping us deal with stress and anxiety is chamomile. It is a valuable ally to have on hand if you have trouble sleeping at night. It is also said to ease menstrual cramps and lower blood pressure while safeguarding the health of your heart.

5. Ginger.

Fiery ginger is an excellent stimulant and well-liked treatment for nausea, including motion sickness and morning sickness. Ginger also helps to boost the immune system, lower inflammation, and soothe sore joints, among many other health benefits.

6. Turmeric.

Turmeric is a powerful anti-inflammatory and a great all-arounder that can help our bodies with a variety of conditions. Curcumin in particular, which protects our cells from oxidative stress, is one of the many antioxidants that are abundant in it. Numerous chronic conditions, including arthritis, Alzheimer's, cardiovascular disease, and liver disease, have shown promise as potential targets for its treatment.

7. Echinacea.

One of the most well-known healing plants for supporting our bodies during the cold and flu season is echinacea. This perennial plant with purple flowers is believed to boost the immune system, making it easier for us to recover from coughs, colds, and sore throats and reducing our risk of getting them in the first place.

8. Ginseng.

TCM experts prize ginseng, which is regarded as a general tonic. The immune system is said to be strengthened, fatigue is said to vanish, and your cardiovascular health is said to be protected. It is also said to give the user energy and strength.

9. Cinnamon.

Delectable cinnamon is a different herb that lowers inflammation and is used to treat many different illnesses. It is a great herb for protecting your cardiovascular health because it has shown promise in assisting with blood sugar management, lowering cholesterol, and lowering blood pressure. It also functions as a natural analgesic.

10. Dandelion.

The last item on our list of healthy foods is the common hedgerow plant known as the dandelion. It contains components that lessen inflammation and safeguard our livers. Additionally used to treat UTIs and lessen bloating is dandelion, a plant that naturally makes you urinate.

What is an Herbalist's Process

The term "herbalist" refers to a person who uses herbal remedies. Despite the fact that some practitioners go by the title of "medical herbalists," they are not medical professionals.

Why Study Herbal Medicine

The underlying cause of illness is sought after by herbalists. The doctor's decision regarding which herbs to use will be influenced by the symptoms or conditions the patient describes during the consultation. They will also perform a clinical examination, paying attention to particular body parts, and write a special prescription. Patients may take a single herbal supplement or a range of herbal dietary supplements.

The following treatments are frequently applied

• Teas.

• liquid or powdered herbal products in capsule form.

• salts to use in the restroom.

• Oils.

• creams and lotions for the body.

Education and training

There is no standardized training or certification program for herbalists because they do not all pursue the same educational path, unlike doctors who attend medical school. In graduate-level clinical herbal medicine programs offered by some universities, students are encouraged to combine conventional herbal medicine with scientifically supported practices.

Other organizations, like the American Herbalist Guild (AHG), offer memberships and certifications. The AHG mandates 400 hours of training and clinical experience before practitioners are eligible to apply for the title of Registered Herbalist.

Herbalists conduct research.

• Human sciences, including physiology, biochemistry, and anatomy.

• Dietary intake.

• Pharmacy dispensing.

• Botany and the science of plants.

• An empirically based botanical study.

Herbalists are able to enroll in educational programs with an emphasis on complementary or alternative medicine. They might also decide to combine formal education with:.

• Therapeutic guidance.

• Actual circumstances.

33

• Intense self-study.

• Conferences, webinars, or workshops in their area of interest.

Why See an Herbalist

Herbalists can be a source of complementary medicine, not a replacement for a physician or mental health expert. A herbalist may be consulted by some people for:

• Therapies without medication.

Using lifestyle suggestions, how to lessen discomfort or stress.

• having trouble falling asleep.

Following are some considerations for using herbal supplements:.

• Ask your doctor's permission before using any herbal remedies. Numerous medications, therapies, and medical conditions do not interact well with herbs and supplements.

• Perform research. Look for a herbalist who is licensed.

• Examine the label. Never take more than the recommended dosage and abide by the directions.

• Be mindful of any negative effects. If you experience nausea, vertigo, or stomach pain, your body may not be responding well.

From ancient times until the 19th century, when the germ theory of disease was developed, herbalism and medicine have had a long and intertwined history. Science-based evidence has served as the foundation for modern medicine since the 19th century. Herbal remedies have largely been replaced in contemporary healthcare by the evidence-based use of pharmaceutical drugs, frequently derived from medicinal plants. Nevertheless, many people still use a variety of conventional or complementary treatments. A significant amount of herbs are frequently used in these systems. Many of the herbs and spices that humans have historically used to season food contain useful medicinal compounds, and using spices with antimicrobial activity in cooking is part of an ancient response to the threat of food-borne pathogens. As a result, the history of herbalism and food history are intertwined.

Prehistory Medicinal plants have been used by humans since before history was recorded. Archaeological evidence suggests that people began using medicinal plants in the Paleolithic, or about 60,000 years ago. Plant samples found in ancient graves have been used to support the idea that Paleolithic people were familiar with herbal medicine (additionally, other non-human primates are known to consume medicinal plants to treat illness). For instance, "Shanidar IV," a 60,000-year-old Neanderthal burial site in northern Iraq, has produced significant amounts of pollen from 8 plant species, 7 of which are currently used as herbal remedies. Paul B. According to Pettitt, a recent analysis of the microfauna from the strata into which the grave was cut suggests that the burrowing rodent Merionestersicus, which is common in the Shanidar microfauna and whose burrowing activity can be observed today, is responsible for depositing the pollen.

The possessions of Tzi the Iceman, whose body was preserved for more than 5,000 years in the Alps of the Tztal, included medicinal herbs. The parasites discovered in his intestines appear to have been treated with these herbs.

History from long ago. The Ebers Papyrus (circa c. A cannabis sativa (marijuana) topical prescription for inflammation dates back to 1550 BCE in ancient Egypt.

Mesopotamia

The Sumerians, who produced clay tablets with lists of hundreds of medicinal plants (including myrrh and opium), are credited with starting the written study of herbs in Mesopotamia more than 5,000 years ago.

Egyptian antiquity The language and translation debates that surround texts from this time and place, specifically ancient Egypt, make them of particular interest. These discrepancies in conclusions result from a lack of thorough understanding of the Egyptian language; many translations are made up of rough approximations between Egyptian and modern concepts, and meaning or context can never be completely certain. Despite the lack of tangible records, texts like the Papyrus Ebers help to clarify and dispel some of the myths surrounding ancient herbal practices. The Papyrus contains descriptions of over 850 plant medicines, including garlic, juniper, cannabis, castor bean, aloe, and mandrake, as well as lists of diseases and their treatments, ranging from "diseases of the limbs" to "diseases of the skin.". The most common symptoms were thought to be the disease itself, so treatments were primarily focused on helping the patient get rid of them. Since many of the texts that are available for translation assume that the doctor already has some knowledge of how treatments are conducted and that such techniques would not need to be reiterated, knowledge of the collection and preparation of such remedies is largely unknown.

There is no doubt that trade and politics spread the Egyptian tradition to regions around the world, influencing and evolving many cultures' medical practices and providing a window into the world of ancient Egyptian medicine. Modern understanding of Egyptian herbals originates from the translation of ancient texts. Although some were imported from other areas, like Lebanon, the majority of the herbs used by Egyptian healers were native to Egypt. Illustrations in tombs or jars with traces of herbs have also been found to provide herbal medicine evidence in addition to papyri.

Rome and Early Greece

Hippocrates

The "Father of Western Medicine," Hippocrates of Kos, is credited with writing a number of texts that make up the Hippocratic Corpus. Each of these texts reflects the broad principles advanced by Hippocrates and his followers, despite the fact that some of these texts' actual authors are in dispute. Parts of the Corpus contain recipes and remedies that undoubtedly reveal common and prevalent treatments from the early ancient Greek era.

Even though the Corpus contains a variety of herbal remedies, none of them are used in religious healing practices, they differ noticeably from them in that they don't involve rituals, prayers, or chants. This distinction demonstrates how the Hippocratics valued reason and logic in medical practice.

Numerous herbs, both native to Greece and those brought in from far-off lands like Arabia, are among the ingredients mentioned in the Corpus. Some of the suggested ingredients include the more accessible and less expensive elderberries and St. John's wort, whereas many imported goods would have been too expensive for everyday household use. It's called John's Wort.

Galen

Galen of Pergamon, a Greek physician who practiced in Rome, was very active in his effort to record his knowledge of all things medical. As part of this endeavor, he wrote numerous texts about herbs and their properties, most notably his Works of Therapeutics. Galen describes how the various medical specialties work together in this text to restore health and fend off disease. Galen's extensive work on the four basic qualities and the humors helped pharmacists better tailor their treatments for each individual patient and their particular symptoms, even though the field of therapeutics covers a wide range of topics.

Carystian Diocles

Diocles of Carystus produced a large number of lengthy writings. His advice on herbalism and treatment was respected enough to earn him the moniker "the second Hippocrates.". Diocles has been quoted extensively throughout history by medical scholars, despite the fact that the original texts no longer exist. It is from these quotations that we learn about his writings. Many of his contemporaries, including Galen, Celsus, and Soranus, are said to have cited Diocles' purportedly first comprehensive herbal, which they credit with being the first complete herbal.

Pliny

Pliny the Elder's Natural History, one of the first encyclopedic works, offers a thorough overview of nature as well as a comprehensive list of medicinal herbs. Pliny's writings offer a vast body of knowledge from which we can glean more information about historical herbalism and medical procedures, with over 900 drugs and plants listed. The greatest of all natural processes, according to Pliny, are illnesses, and the use of drugs to treat them has an effect on the "state of peace or of war which exists between the various departments of nature.".

Dioscorides

Similar to Pliny, Pedanius Dioscorides created a pharmacopeia called De Materia Medica that included over 1000 drugs made from herbs, minerals, and animals. The remedies included in this work were frequently used in antiquity, and Dioscorides was the foremost authority on medicines for more than 1,600 years.

Theophrastus' HistoriaPlantarum, written in the fourth century BC, which was the first systematization of the botanical world, was equally significant for herbalists and botanists of later centuries.

The Middle Ages

Medical care in the Islamic world of the middle ages.

Although there are texts from the medieval era that clearly indicate the uses of herbs, there has been much debate among scholars about the actual reasons for and understandings behind the creation of herbal documents during this time. According to the first point of view, these medieval texts' information was simply copied verbatim from their classical counterparts without much consideration or understanding. The second argument, which is gaining support from contemporary academics, contends that copies of herbals were made with real-world use in mind and were supported by genuine understanding.

The majority of the knowledge of plants, plant names, and plant lore that medical writers and students of medicine had in the fifth century was based on the classical texts and practices. Greek or Latin was the common language in the majority of classical botanical texts. The Greeks and Romans eventually studied herbalism when it eventually became a subfield of modern medicine. In order to document and comprehend the history of herbalism that spanned many centuries, they had to transition their knowledge of these significant medicinal plants. Herbalists in the fifth to tenth centuries encountered problems because they lacked knowledge of the subject because it had not yet been discovered and thoroughly studied. Western Europe's first century BC is when herbalism is first mentioned. In addition to being essential for surviving in the Middle Ages without modern prescription drugs, herbalism served as the foundation for the natural remedies we still use today. Since the Stone Age, people have been aware of the practice of herbalism. The development of medicine throughout history has been greatly influenced by plant medicine.

The inclusion of numerous plant chapters, symptom lists, habitat details, and plant synonyms in texts like the Herbarium is some evidence that herbals were used with knowledge.

Some notable texts used during this time period include Bald's Leechbook, the Lacnunga, the perididaxeon, Herbarium Apulei, De Taxone, and Medicina de Quadrupedibus; however, the Ex Herbis Femininis, the Herbarius, and works by

Dioscorides were the most widely read. In the year 50 AD, a Greek physician and botanist named Dioscorides devoted his entire life to learning about plants and how to use their therapeutic properties. Dioscoride's writings were the main source of information about plants and how to use their properties during the Middle Ages.

Dioscorides was fortunate enough to have writing abilities, and because of his travels, studies, and writings about herbalism, he is a significant figure in herbalism. These texts, known as "De materia medica," were originally composed in five volumes in Greek and were later translated into Latin by Dioscorides. Dioscorides' writings are significant because they represent the first written account of herbalism from the fifth century, and at that time in western Europe, this text served as the foundation for all subsequent knowledge. The herbal medical documents offered enough details about herbs, their appearances, and their applications.

The Middle East and Asia, where Discordies frequently traveled for research purposes to carry out fresh studies on herbalism, are where the majority of our knowledge about these regions comes from. He wrote about numerous other foreign herbs and plants that originated in Asia while conducting his research. This made a significant contribution to trade in Europe between the early fifth and the tenth centuries, as well as to the expanding field of herbalism.

Dioscorides was intrigued by these various herbs because he had never seen them before and because of their healing properties. This gave him the idea that these herbs might have a new impact on natural medicine. He learned about the spice trade, also known as the trade in dried herbs, when he visited the West. During the Middle Ages, herbalists came together extensively as a result of Dioscorides' writing of these medical texts.

The southern regions of Europe, including Italy and Greece, were where the plants grew the best. The fact that these herbs could not only be found closer to the sea than they were on land gives them a special quality.

It was challenging to have specific knowledge about these herbs and their beneficial properties in the early fifth century without documentation. Discordies volumes gave information on the characteristics of poisonous plants, their geographic range, and useful cautions.

A lot of herbalists were unaware of how important it was to remember that some herbs could only grow in specific regions. Due to the lack of socioeconomic or climatic factors in that area, certain herbs with medicinal properties had to be traded, which is why the spice trade played a significant role in the development of medicine during the medieval era. Scholars who were not familiar with plants that grew in other regions would gain a great deal from this. Each plant was identified, and Dioscorides' writing and knowledge of his volumes described its characteristics, application, and color.

Citrus, ginger, echinacea, and goldenseal are a few examples of non-Western herbs and plants. These specimens were unique to Asia and were not indigenous to nations like Britain. Despite the fact that these herbs and plants were grown and indigenous to Asia, the use of spices made many Eastern herbs and plants important and gave herbalists access to new information.

Elderberry, wild sage, rosehips, plantain, calendula, comfrey, yarrow, nettle, and many other herbs were among the most important ones that were used in the Middle Ages. Similar to how natural remedies like calming teas and ointments are used today to treat minor injuries and colds, each of these herbs has unique properties that herbalists used to treat their patients. The origins of the recipe are from medieval herbalists, though the ingredients may be changed.

The majority of the herbs that were collected and used during the Middle Ages were wild-grown, which refers to herbs that were taken directly from the earth, unprocessed, and without cultivation. To see the results of their beneficial properties, those that were studied would undergo some processing.

The local population could access the kinds of herbs that typically grew in the wild, so herbalism was not just a subject dominated by academics. Herbalists discovered not only the use of plants grown in the wild, but also the use of natural plants that were used as drugs for major operations or for psychoactive purposes. Before being imported to nations like Italy, France, and Great Britain, cannabis was first sold in Egypt. When people discovered that cannabis could treat anxiety, pain, and other ailments, its use increased.

Opioids were also employed by herbalists as painkillers. Herbalists used plants not only for minor ailments and wounds, but also for drugs, major operations, and psychoactive purposes. Herb use in various forms increased during the late Middle Ages in the 10th century. The use of essential oils, ointments, and other products from herbalism only became more popular after the 10th century. Both for daily use and for the treatment of illness, these new types of medications were used.

During the Early Middle Ages, the main repository of medical knowledge in Europe and England was the Benedictine monasteries. However, instead of developing significant new knowledge and practices, these monastic scholars spent the majority of their time translating and copying works from ancient Arabic and Greco-Roman cultures.

Numerous Greek and Roman writings on medicine, as well as writings on other topics, were copied by hand in monasteries. Thus, the monasteries tended to develop into regional hubs of medical learning, and their herb gardens supplied the essential ingredients for straightforward treatment of common ailments. Hildegard of Bingen was one of the most well-known women in the herbal tradition. CausaeetCurae was authored by a Benedictine nun from the 12th century. Herbalism at this time was primarily practiced by women, especially in Germanic tribes. At the same time, folk medicine continued unabatedly in the home and village, providing employment for numerous roving and permanent herbalists. Among them were the "wise-women" and "wise men," who frequently offered advice, spells, enchantments, and herbal remedies.

The three foremost authorities on healing at the time were the Arabian School, Anglo-Saxon leechcraft, and Salerno. The Canon of Medicine, which Avicenna wrote, became the main source of medical knowledge in the Arab world. He was a great scholar of the Arabian School. The Canon of Medicine is renowned for its introduction of methodical experimentation and the study of physiology, the discovery of infectious diseases and sexually transmitted diseases, the introduction of quarantine to stop the spread of infectious diseases, the introduction of experimental medicine, clinical trials, and the idea of a syndrome in the diagnosis of particular diseases. dot. The Canon includes descriptions of about 760 medicinal plants and the potential medications that can be made from them. Leech was the English word for doctor, but it also made me think of some of their treatments, so I called it WithLeechcraft. With a focus on health and medicine, Salerno was a renowned center for higher education. The school was attended by Constantine the African, who is credited with bringing Arabic medicine to Europe.

Herbs in a Universal Language

The key concept is herbal.

In the Middle Ages, a critical examination of plant science began. The 16th and 17th centuries saw a revival of interest in botany in Europe, which eventually spread to America as a result of European conquest and colonization.

Philosophers started using herbs, and academics studied a lot of different kinds of plants.

Herbalists first focused on medicinal applications before turning their attention to plant uses in agriculture and food production. Herbalists, also referred to as botanists in the Middle Ages, gathered, raised, dried, stored, and sketched plants. The ability to categorize and identify plants based on their morphology, habitats, and usefulness was cultivated by many. These books, referred to as herbals, contained descriptions of how to use various plants along with beautiful paintings and illustrations of those plants.

In both botany and gardening at the time, the importance of plants for humans' needs was emphasized; the well-known herbal also covered these uses. Throughout the Middle Ages, book culture grew and eventually spread throughout the entire medieval world. The phenomenon of translation has a long history, dating back to the eighth century in Baghdad, where it began as an academic pursuit, and spreading by the eleventh and twelfth centuries to other academic centers in the Mediterranean region.

It takes a lot of people working together to translate something.

How people in the Middle Ages viewed nature, however, is unknown.

Different versions and compilations of particular manuscripts from various sources, both old and new, have been created through text and image translation. The dynamic process of translation, which also served as a significant academic endeavor, was responsible for the significant scientific advancements of the Middle Ages. It was well known that the Benedictine monasteries had a thorough understanding of herbs. Since these gardens grew the herbs that were believed to be effective in treating the various human ills, monastic influence can be traced to the origins of modern medical education. establishing monastic universities and teaching monks how to translate Greek manuscripts into Latin.

Botanical knowledge was closely related to medical knowledge because in the middle ages, remedies were the main use of the plant. The names of the plants, distinguishing traits, medicinal plant parts, therapeutic properties, and in some cases even usage instructions were used to organize the herbals. To use herbal remedies effectively in medicine, a manual had to be written. Dioscorides' De material medica was a significant herbal that was written for everyday use.

Theophrastus described the characteristics of more than 500 plants in more than 200 papers. He developed a classification scheme for plants based on their morphology, which covers form and structure. Regarding pepper, cinnamon, bananas, asparagus, and cotton, he went into great detail. His best-known works, Enquiry into Plants and The Causes of Plants, were both translated into Latin and have remained influential for many centuries. He has been referred to as the "grandfather of botany.".

Crateuas was the first to write a book on the pharmacology of medicinal plants, and his work had a long-lasting impact on medicine. Greek physician Pedanius Dioscorides wrote more than 600 descriptions of various plant species' therapeutic properties. Even during the Renaissance, pharmacology and medicine used his illustrations.

Medical facilities have become established in monasteries. Both monks and their patients received information on these herbal remedies and how to use them. For those who already knew about and could comprehend herbal remedies, these complicated illustrations would be useless. It has been questioned whether these herbal remedies are actually helpful because several plants are portrayed as claiming to treat the same condition and because "the modern world does not like such impression.". When utilized by qualified healers, as stated in ", these plants can be used for a variety of purposes.

These medieval healers didn't need any assistance in choosing their plants because their training had equipped them to treat a wide range of medical conditions. The monks gathered and arranged texts with the intention of using them in their monasteries. Medieval monks changed a lot of treatments for both their own needs and the needs of the neighborhood. This may be the cause of the partial incompatibility of the current treatment collections.

Another translation technique used to transfer medical knowledge from one generation to the next was oral transmission. While it's a common misconception that one can learn about early medieval medicine by simply identifying texts, it can be difficult to put together a thorough understanding of herbals without prior knowledge. The act of writing or illustrating was only a small part of what influenced the translation of these herbals; instead, these remedies are the result of numerous previous translations that combined knowledge from numerous influences.

Early modern
When many of them were made available for the first time in languages other than Latin or Greek, the 16th and 17th centuries are considered the golden age of herbals. The use of plants from the Americas increased during the 18th and 19th centuries, during which time modern medicine was also developed.

The 16th century

The first English-language herbal was printed in 1526, under the pseudonym Grete Herball. The two most well-known herbals in English are Nicholas Culpeper's The English Physician Enlarged (1653) and John Gerard's The Herball or General History of Plants (1597). Gerard essentially translated works by the Belgian herbalist Dodoens into his text and illustrations. The first edition contained a number of errors as a result of the two parts' improper assembly. Although Culpeper's integration of traditional medicine with astrology, magic, and folklore was ridiculed by the doctors of the day, his book, like Gerard's and other herbals, was incredibly popular. The Columbian Exchange and the Age of Exploration saw the introduction of new medicinal plants to Europe. The Badianus Manuscript is a Nahuatl and Latin-written 16th-century illustrated Mexican herbal.

18th century

However, the second millennium also saw the start of a gradual decline in the dominant position held by plants as sources of therapeutic effects. The Black Death, which the then-dominant Four Element medical system was unable to stop, marked the beginning of this. Arsenic, copper sulfate, iron, mercury, and sulfur are just a few examples of the active chemical drugs that Paracelsus popularized a century later.

Nineteenth century

With doctors being few and far between in the Americas, herbalists were the primary source of medical knowledge. These books included encyclopedias, Buchan's Domestic Medicine, Dodoens' New Herbal, Edinburgh New Dispensatory, and other works. Native Americans also shared some of their knowledge with colonists in addition to Europeans' knowledge of American plants, but the majority of these records were not written and compiled until the 19th century. John Bartram was a botanist who researched the treatments that Native Americans would divulge and frequently included tidbits of information about these plants in printed almanacs.

Understanding of the precise effects that drugs have on the body has improved since pharmacology was formalized in the 19th century. Samuel Thompson, an untrained but well-respected herbalist at the time, had such an impact on medical and herbalist thinking that people today still refer to Thompsonians as his followers. They stood out from the "regular" physicians of the day who practiced bloodletting and calomel, and they helped to spark a brief revival of herbal medicine's empirical approach.

Current time

Since the Flexner Report of 1910, which caused the closure of the eclectic medical schools where only botanical medicine was taught, traditional herbalism has been regarded as an alternative medical practice in the United States. Traditional Chinese medicine, which made extensive use of herbalism, was once again incorporated into China's healthcare system in 1949 by Mao Zedong. Since then, schools have been instructing thousands of practitioners—including Americans—in the fundamentals of Chinese medicine for use in hospitals. While herbalism was causing controversy in Britain in the 1930s, government regulation started to forbid it in the United States.

80 percent of people worldwide, according to the World Health Organization, rely on herbal remedies for some aspect of their primary healthcare. About 70% of German doctors prescribe

one of the 600–700 plant-based medications that are readily available there.

In the United States, it is legal to prescribe treatments and cures to patients with the help of a medical license, which is granted at the state level. No state currently requires anyone to obtain a license or certification as an herbalist in order to use, sell, or recommend herbs.

"Traditional medicine is a complex network of interconnected theories and practices, requiring a multidisciplinary approach to study. The diverse abilities of plants and their lack of harmful side effects have led many alternative doctors in the twenty-first century to incorporate herbalism in traditional medicine.

What Advantages Do Herbal Medicines Offer

Many of us want to try a drug that won't cause more harm than good because we have encountered side effects from conventional medications. Others prefer a more natural approach to treatment because it makes them feel more secure to know that their medication is derived from nature and functions in harmony with the body rather than in opposition to it.

Herbal medicine: What is it

Herbal medicine, also known as herbalism or botanical medicine, uses plants and their extracts to treat a wide range of medical conditions. Herbal medicine promotes health without the negative side effects associated with conventional therapies by utilizing the power of nature.

What distinguishes conventional medicine from herbal medicine?

Herbal remedies work with the body to reestablish balance, as opposed to traditional medications, which only address symptoms and sometimes worsen the condition.

Herbal medicine works in harmony with your body to improve health, unlike conventional medicine, which can make the body's balance worse. People without access to conventional medicine use herbal remedies to treat themselves all over the world, and many more use herbal remedies that are sold in stores.

Do not forget that the efficacy and purity of herbal medicines can vary.

Depression

Without being aware of it, many people use echinacea as an immune stimulant. Although science has only recently begun to investigate many of the beneficial compounds found in herbal medicines, herbal medicine practitioners have long known about them.

What Conditions Are Treatable with Herbal Medicine

There are a number of conditions that herbal medicine can treat orimprove:

Herbal medicine will typically be suggested as a component of a treatment plan that also includes dietary and lifestyle changes, supplements, and extra nutrients. It may be time to think about consulting an herbal medicine practitioner who takes a more balanced and holistic approach, as traditional doctors frequently have no effective treatment for these conditions or only offer a treatment that seems as bad as the disease.

Advantages of Herbal Medicine

For ages, herbal medicine has been regarded as a trustworthy form of treatment. or, at the very least, 60,000 years according to archaeological evidence. Currently, according to the

World Health Organization, 25% of the global population uses herbs for basic healthcare. While it falls under the umbrella of complementary medicine, it is deeply entwined with attaining the highest level of overall wellbeing, healing, and holistic preventative action. If these advantages are properly utilized, the ripple effects could be life-altering. The key advantages of using herbal medicine are listed below.

Affordable and reachable

A certified naturopath should always prescribe high quality herbs in controlled dosages. Although this is (for reputable naturopaths) somewhat of a myth, some people may view this step as an expensive barrier to obtaining herbs. A more cost-effective alternative for herbal medicine is to visit a naturopath since most general practitioners no longer offer the option of bulk billing. The right herbs can help with disease prevention, ongoing health and wellbeing, and disease treatments. Herbs can have extremely high efficacy in relatively low dosages, either by themselves or in combination with medications (which must always be disclosed to your naturopath). So for a relatively low price point, a little goes a long way. Effective herbs will also ensure that you visit your GP and naturopath much less frequently.

Healing through natural means
Herbs are an entirely natural method of treatment, prevention, and health

promotion. They are a safe and effective alternative to, or supplement to, some pharmacy medications when used as directed and individually prescribed for your needs. Herbal medicines can be a valuable addition to your holistic health regimen, and when used properly, there are very few, if any, drawbacks.

Reduced Danger of Adverse Effects
Contrary to many prescription drugs, using herbal medicine as directed results in significantly fewer side effects. They use formulations that are intended to continuously support and fortify the body. They have significantly fewer instances of severe reactions, dependency, and complications despite having a high efficacy. You won't experience crippling

comedowns if you decide to stop using herbal remedies; at most, you might notice the return of the symptoms you were trying to get rid of with the herbs, but not at a higher intensity. .

Different herbs can be tested and used safely

High quality natural medicinal herbs can be tested and trialed in a safe manner with little downtime if done so under the direction of a qualified professional. While we might ask you to wait a certain amount of time before trying another herb, this is usually done to better gauge how and whether it is working for you.

How to Use Herbs Effortlessly and Safely

These ideas about herbs will help you understand how safe—or dangerous—any herb might be.

Are herbs "dilute forms of drugs" and therefore dangerous? Or are they "natural" and therefore safe? It depends on the herb.

To avoid issues when purchasing or using herbs, take the following four steps:

Using the "wrong" herb is one of the simplest ways to get into trouble when using them. Common names for herbs overlap, leading to confusion as to their correct identity. Even herbs with accurate labels sometimes have extraneous parts from other, more harmful herbs. Herbs may be harvested at the incorrect time or handled improperly after harvesting, causing them to acquire negative traits.

If you grow the herbs you sell, take great care to harvest and dry each plant separately, and be meticulous with labeling. Only purchase herbs from reliable vendors.

Buying herbs should only be done if they are marked with their botanical name. Even though common names for plants can apply to a variety of plants, botanical names are specific. Both Tagetes, an annual used as a bedding plant, and Calendula officinalis, a medicinal herb, can be used to describe "marigold.".

Simply put, use one herb at a time.

One herb is one simple. I prepare, buy, sell, teach about, and use herbal simples—preparations made from just one herb—for maximum safety. (On occasion, I flavor a remedy by adding some mint.

The likelihood of unpleasant side effects increases with the number of herbs in a formula. It makes sense that people look for combinations in order to get more for their money. And a lot of people are under the impression that herbs must be combined in order to be effective (possibly because potentially poisonous herbs are frequently combined with protective herbs to lessen the damage they cause). However, combining herbs with similar properties, such as goldenseal and echinacea, is counterproductive and more likely to result in problems than a simple. Echinacea tincture alone is much safer and more efficient than any combination.

All substances, including drugs, foods, and herbs, cause different reactions in various people. It is impossible to pinpoint which herb is to blame when several herbs are combined in a formula and someone who consumes it experiences unpleasant side effects. Simples make it simple to identify which herb is performing which function. Other herbs with related properties can be tried if there is a negative reaction. Additional protection is provided by keeping the number of herbs consumed per day (to no more than four).

Herbal side effects are typically milder and less frequent than drug side effects. It's possible that the body is still learning how to process an herb if it upsets digestion. Before giving up, give it a few more tries. Any herb that makes you feel sick, queasy, or gives you severe stomach pains, diarrhea, a headache, or blurred vision should be stopped. These effects usually take place fairly quickly. (Slippery elm is a superb antidote for any poison.

It is especially important to consult resources that list the side effects of herbs before using them if you have allergies to any foods or medications.

The effectiveness of the same herb varies depending on how it is prepared.

Any herbal remedy's safety depends on how it is made and used.

Alkaloids, or plant parts that are poisonous, are present in tinctures and extracts, so they must be used with caution and discretion. Tinctures are as safe as the herb they contain (for tonifying, stimulating, sedating, or potentially toxic herbs, see the warnings below). In particular when using powerful herbs, simples should be used or sold rather than combinations.

Particularly when nourishing or tonifying herbs are used, dried herbs made into teas or infusions contain the nourishing elements of the plants and are generally quite safe.

The least effective way to use herbs is typically in dried herb capsules. They are expensive, poorly utilized, frequently stale or ineffective, and poorly digested.

Herbal oils that have been infused with other substances can be purchased unthickened or as ointments. They are much less dangerous than essential oils, which are extremely concentrated and dangerous if consumed internally.

Herbal vinegars are rich in minerals in addition to being aesthetically pleasing. An excellent vehicle for nourishing and tonifying herbs; not as potent as tinctures for stimulants/sedatives.

Those who prefer to avoid alcohol can purchase herbal glycerins, but they typically have a weaker effect than tinctures.

Be careful when using poisonous, stimulating, tonifying, and nourishing herbs.

Several thousand plants with widely varying functions make up the category of herbs. Some are potential poisons, some are nourishing, some are tonifying, some are stimulants and sedatives. To use them wisely and effectively, we must comprehend each category, its applications, the best way to prepare them, and the typical dosage range.

The safest herbs are those that nourish; adverse effects are extremely uncommon. Herbs that nourish the body can be consumed in any quantity for any period of time. Like spinach and kale, they are consumed as food. High concentrations of essential fatty acids, antioxidants, carotenes, vitamins, minerals, and proteins can be found in nourishing herbs. Alfalfa, amaranth, astragalus, calendula blossoms, comfrey leaves, chickweed, honeysuckle flowers, lamb's quarter, marshmallow, nettles, oatstraw, plantain (leaves/seeds), purslane, red clover blossoms, seaweed, Siberian ginseng, slippery elm, violet leaves, and wild mushrooms are some examples of nourishing herbs.

Tonifying herbs work gradually in the body and have a cumulative effect as opposed to an immediate one. They increase an organ's or a system's capacity to function, such as the immune system or the liver. When used sparingly and continuously for a long time, tonifying herbs are most effective. Less is required the more bitter the tonic tastes. As with nourishing herbs, bland tonics can be used liberally.

Tonics occasionally cause side effects, but they are typically very transient. Older herbalists frequently confused stimulating and tonifying herbs, which resulted in widespread herb misuse and harmful side effects. Ground ivy, hawthorn berries, horsetail, lady's mantle, lemon balm, milk thistle seeds, motherwort, mullein, paud'arco, raspberry leaves, schisandra berries, St. John's wort, and crone(mug)wort are some examples of tonifying herbs. Joan's wort, yellow dock, usnea, turmeric root, and wild yam.

Herbs that are sedating or stimulating can produce a range of swift reactions, some of which may be undesirable. Some aspects of the person might experience stress in order to support other aspects. No matter if they are herbal or synthetic, strong sedatives and stimulants force us to act outside of our normal ranges of activity and may have severe side effects. If we rely on them and then try to function without them, we end up more agitated (or depressed) than when we started. Regular consumption of potent sedatives and stimulants, such as opium, rhubarb root, cayenne, or coffee, causes loss of tone, functional impairment, and even physical dependence. The dose must be moderate and the duration of use must be reduced the stronger the herb.

Some of my favorite herbs are those that sooth and nourish while sedating or stimulating. They do not lead to dependency, so I use them freely. sedative/stimulant herbs that also tonify or nourish: boneset, catnip, citrus peel, cleavers, ginger, hops, lavender, marjoram, motherwort, oatstraw, passion flower, peppermint, rosemary, sage, skullcap.

Angelica, Black pepper, licorice, coffee, blessed thistle root, cayenne, cinnamon, and opium are some of the other ingredients, poppies, osha root, shepherd's purse, sweet woodruff, turkey rhubarb root, uvaursu leaves, valerian root, wild lettuce sap, willow bark, and wintergreen leaves are among the herbs that have strong sedative/stimulant properties.

Potentially lethal herbs are intense, potent medicines that are used sparingly and only as long as necessary. Common side effects are present. The following herbs are some examples of those that could be poisonous: belladonna, blood-root, celandine, chaparral, foxglove, goldenseal, henbane, iris root, Jimson weed, lobelia, May apple (American mandrake), mistletoe, poke root, poison hemlock, stillingia root, turkey corn root, and wild cucumber root.

Think about the following ideas as you use herbs safely:

- Recognize the potent influence plants have on the body and the spirit.

- By using herbal remedies for minor or external issues prior to or concurrently with working on major and internal issues, you can increase your faith in the ability of plants to heal

- Get to know knowledgeable healers who are interested in herbal medicine and maintain relationships with them, either in person or through books

- Embrace the individuality of each and every plant, person, and circumstance.

- Keep in mind that everyone heals and becomes whole at their own rate and in their own particular way. This process can be aided by people, animals, and plants
- However, the healing is carried out by the body and spirit
- Not all ailments can be cured by plants

The Top 9 Herbal Medicines in the World

1. Echinacea

A flowering plant known as coneflower or echinacea is a well-known herbal remedy.

Native Americans in North America have long used this plant, which is native to that continent, to treat a wide range of illnesses, including stomach upset, toothaches, burns, wounds, and burns.

The plant's leaves, petals, roots, and other parts can all be used medicinally, but many people think the roots have the most potent impact.

Echinacea can be applied topically in addition to being typically consumed as a tea or supplement.

Though the science supporting this isn't all that compelling, it is now primarily used to treat or prevent the common cold.

Echinacea may reduce the risk of getting a cold by 10 to 20 percent when taken, according to one study involving more than 4,000 people but there is scant to no evidence that it can treat a cold once you have one.

Although there is not enough information to assess this herb's effects over the long term, short-term use is typically regarded as safe. Though occasionally reported side effects include nauseousness, stomach discomfort, and skin

The majority of supermarkets and health food stores carry echinacea, but you can also order it online.

SUMMARY

A flowering plant called echinacea is frequently used to both treat and prevent the common cold. Despite the limited research, it may up to 20% lower your chance of getting a cold.

2. Ginseng

Ginseng is a medicinal plant whose roots are usually steeped to make a tea or dried to make a powder.

It is frequently used in traditional Chinese medicine to bolster immunity, brain function, and energy levels while reducing inflammation.

There are numerous varieties, but the two most well-known kinds are the American and Asian varieties, Panaxquinquefolius and Panax ginseng, respectively. The relaxing effects of American ginseng are thought to outweigh the stimulating effects of Asian ginseng.

Despite being used for centuries, ginseng's effectiveness has not been adequately studied in the modern era.

Its distinctive compounds, known as ginsenosides, are thought to possess neuroprotective, anticancer, antidiabetic, and immune-supportive properties, according to numerous test-tube and animal studies.

Human research is nevertheless required

Ginseng is regarded as relatively safe for short-term use, but its long-term safety is unknown.

Headaches, insufficient sleep, and digestive problems are examples of possible side effects.

The majority of health food stores carry ginseng, and it is also available online.

SUMMARY

In traditional Chinese medicine, ginseng is a herbal supplement frequently used to increase energy, brain function, and resistance to disease.

However, there aren't enough human studies.

3. Ginkgo blatt

Ginkgo biloba, also referred to as ginkgo, is a herbal remedy made from maidenhair trees.

Ginkgo biloba is a tree that is native to China and has been used for thousands of years in traditional Chinese medicine. It is still one of the most popular herbal supplements available today. It has a number of strong antioxidants in it that are thought to have several advantages.

The seeds and leaves are traditionally used to create teas and tinctures, but leaf extract is used in the majority of contemporary applications.

The uncooked fruit and toasted seeds are also favored by some people. However, the seeds should only be consumed in small amounts, if at all, as they are only mildly toxic.

Heart disease, dementia, mental health issues, and sexual dysfunction are just a few of the maladies that ginkgo is said to treat.

However, research hasn't shown it to be efficient for any of these issues

Most people tolerate it well, but there could be some side effects, such as headache, heart palpitations, digestive problems, skin reactions, and an elevated risk of bleeding

Ginkgo can be purchased online or at supplement stores.

SUMMARY

Although gingko has historically been used to treat a wide range of conditions, such as heart disease, dementia, and sexual dysfunction, contemporary research has not yet established the effectiveness of this use for any of these conditions.

4. Elderberry

The cooked fruit of the Sambucusnigra plant is typically used to make elderberry, an age-old herbal remedy. It has long been used to treat constipation, colds, viral infections, toothaches, headaches, and nerve pain.

Nowadays, the product is marketed primarily as a remedy for cold and flu symptoms.

There is no established dosage for elderberry, but it can be purchased as a syrup or lozenge. Some people favor cooking elderberries with additional ingredients like honey and ginger to create their own syrup or tea.

Although human research is lacking, test-tube studies show that its plant compounds have antioxidant, antimicrobial, and antiviral.

Elderberry appears to shorten the duration of flu infections in a few small human, but larger studies are required to determine whether it is any more effective than standard antiviral medications.

Although unripe or raw fruit is toxic and can cause symptoms like nausea, vomiting, and diarrhea, short-term use is thought to be safe.

When you next visit a health store, keep an eye out for this herbal remedy or purchase it online.

SUMMARY

Elderberry is used to treat the symptoms of the common cold and the flu, and some research indicates that it may be at least marginally effective. Elderberry is toxic if consumed unripe or raw, but it is safe when cooked.

5. St. It's called John's wort

St. Hypericumperforatum, a flowering plant, is the source of the herbal remedy known as St. John's wort (SJW). Teas, capsules, and extracts are frequently made from its tiny, yellow flowers.

SJW has been used since the time of ancient Greece, and in some regions of Europe, doctors continue to frequently prescribe it.

In the past, it was used to promote wound healing, treat depression and various kidney and lung diseases as well as to relieve insomnia. Today, mild to moderate depression is primarily treated with this medication.

Numerous studies have found that short-term SJW use is just as effective as some common antidepressants. For those with severe depression or suicidal thoughts, there isn't much information on long-term safety or effectiveness Although SJW has few adverse effects, it can cause allergic reactions, light sensitivity, confusion, dizziness, and dry mouth.

Numerous medications, such as birth control, blood thinners, some painkillers, antidepressants, and some cancer treatments, are also affected by it.

If you take any prescription drugs, talk to your doctor before using SJW because certain drug interactions can be fatal.

SJW is accessible online and in many stores if you decide to give it a try.

SUMMARY

St. John's wort can be used to treat light to moderate depression. However, because it interacts with a number of conventional medicines, you might need to use caution or avoid it.

6. Turmeric

An herb that is a member of the ginger family is turmeric (Curcuma longa).

It has been used for thousands of years in both cooking and medicine, but only recently has its potent anti-inflammatory power come to light.

The primary active ingredient in turmeric is curcumin. Numerous conditions, such as anxiety, metabolic syndrome, chronic pain, and inflammation may all be treated by it.

More precisely, numerous studies demonstrate that supplemental doses of curcumin are equally effective at reducing arthritis pain as some well-known anti-inflammatory medications, such as ibuprofen. Both turmeric and curcumin supplements are generally regarded as safe, but very high doses may result in diarrhea, headaches, or skin irritation.

You can also use fresh or dried turmeric in dishes like curries, though it is unlikely that the amount you typically eat in food will have a significant medicinal effect.

Consider purchasing supplements online instead.

SUMMARY

Because of its well-known anti-inflammatory effects, turmeric may be especially useful in treating arthritis pain.

7. Ginger

Ginger is a popular herb that is also used as a remedy. Although it can be eaten fresh or dried, the tea and capsules are the main medicinal forms.

Similar to turmeric, ginger also grows underground as a rhizome. As a result of the beneficial compounds it contains, it has been used for a long time in both traditional and modern medicine to treat conditions like high blood pressure, nausea, migraines, and colds.

Its best-known contemporary application is the management of nausea associated with chemotherapy, pregnancy, and surgical procedures.

Though the evidence is contradictory, research on animals and in test tubes also suggests potential benefits for treating and preventing diseases like cancer and heart disease.

Some small human studies have suggested that this root might reduce your risk of developing blood clots, despite not having been proven to be any more effective than conventional treatments.

Ginger is largely tolerated by most people.

Although adverse side effects are rare, high doses may cause mild diarrhea or heartburn.

Online and in your local supermarket are both places to find supplements for ginger.

SUMMARY

Although ginger is most commonly used to treat nausea, it also contains a number of strong plant compounds that can be used to treat a variety of conditions.

8. Valerian

The flowering plant known as valerian, also known as "nature's Valium," is thought to encourage calmness and tranquility.

114

You can drink valerian root tea or take the dried root as a supplement.

Ancient Greeks and Romans used it to treat headaches, trembling, heart palpitations, and restlessness. It is now most frequently used to treat insomnia and anxiety.

The evidence supporting these uses isn't very strong, though

One analysis discovered valerian to be somewhat effective at promoting sleep despite the fact that many of the study's conclusions were based on participants' subjective reports.

Valerian is generally regarded as safe, despite the possibility that it could cause headaches and digestive issues. If you're taking any other sedatives, you shouldn't take it because there could be additive effects, such as excessive malaise and drowsiness.

Find this herb by doing an online search or visiting various health food stores.

SUMMARY

Valerian root is frequently employed as a natural sleep aid and anxiety treatment despite the lack of strong evidence for its efficacy.

9. Chamomile

The flowering plant chamomile is one of the most well-known herbal remedies in the world.

Even though the dried leaves can also be used to make tea, therapeutic extracts, or topically applied compresses, it's the flowers that are most frequently used to make tea.

Since ancient times, chamomile has been used to treat wounds, urinary tract infections, and infections of the upper respiratory tract. It is also used to treat nausea and stomach pain.

There are more than 100 active compounds in this herb, many of which are thought to be the source of its numerous benefits.

Numerous in vitro and animal studies have demonstrated the anti-inflammatory, antimicrobial, and antioxidant activity of these compounds, but insufficient human research has been done.

Nevertheless, a few small human studies suggest that chamomile can help with diarrhea, emotional issues, cramping from premenstrual syndrome (PMS), and pain and inflammation from osteoarthritis.

Despite the fact that chamomile is generally safe, some people may have an allergic reaction, especially if they have a plant allergy to daisies, ragweed, or marigolds.

The majority of supermarkets and the internet both carry it.

SUMMARY

Chamomile is still one of the most popular herbal medicines in the world and is used to treat a wide range of illnesses despite having little scientific backing.

- use herbal remedies with extreme caution.
- It is best to consult a health expert before considering taking herbal supplements in order to ensure proper dosage, understand potential side effects, and be aware

of interactions with other medications

Safety

It's a common misconception that because herbal medicines are derived from plants, they are inherently safe.

Similar to conventional drugs, herbal supplements can cause serious side effects or interact poorly with other medications you are taking.